I'm safe, Now what?

10 Strategies to get over an Abusive Relationship and take your life back

by Gigi Rosa

**Copyright © 2018 by G.D.R.
All Right Reserved.**

No part of this publication may be reproduced, distributed, or transmitted in any form or by any means, including photocopying, recording, or other electronic or mechanical methods, or by any information storage and retrieval system without the prior written permission of the publisher, except in the case of very brief quotations embodied in critical reviews and certain other noncommercial uses permitted by copyright law.

Table of Contents

Introduction 4

Why I Wrote This Book 5

Chapter 1.   Do not go back 6

Chapter 2. It all starts with a plan 8

    How not to fail 15

Chapter 3. How to stay safe 19

Chapter 4. You can't do this alone 26

    How to find your support team 29

Chapter 5. How to beat your number one enemy 31

    Strategies to overcome this enemy 33

    Affirmations 38

Chapter 6. Get your finances in order 39

    If you have income or savings 39

    Nine ways to get cash if you have no income or savings ... 40

Chapter 7. How to get back on your feet, fast 51

Chapter 8. Why being alone is good for you now 63

Chapter 9. Control this emotion so you can finally move on 67

Chapter 10. Never stop doing this 73

Chapter 11. Retrain your brain 78

About The Author 84

    One Last Thing 85

Introduction

One of the most painful and confusing time in my life was right after I left my abuser. I was extremely hurt, sad and depressed; I didn't know what to do with myself. I felt lonely, weak, and abandoned. Did I make the right decision? How could this happen to me? I was missing him and I hated him. I wasn't sure if I was going to be able to stay away.

There is a roller coaster of emotions that plague your judgment, and this is when most victims go back. Because they don't pause and believe that they are strong, that they deserve better, that they don't have to stay in a toxic relationship for anyone, even the kids.

This book will take you from the day you leave your abuser until you are ready to go on your own and explore what's next for you.

There will be practical advice to get you over the hump and start making some real progress in your life. Every chapter is filled with real life tips and tricks that you can use today to help you make the change.

Every chapter will bring you a complete lesson complete with tools to help you succeed in getting your life back on track. You can skip to any section as you will find a complete lesson on its own, but I do recommend you follow along in the journey so that you can get a complete picture of what you need to do now.

There is no better time like the present to start living your best life. Let's get to work.

Why I Wrote This Book

I looked for books that would speak to me and my current situation; feeling lost and defeated after leaving an abusive relationship. I didn't want to know "why he did that", or how to "understand" a narcissist and abuser. I knew why he did that (he was evil), and how (I had the bruises to prove it).

What I wanted to know was how I could get better, how I could move on and make something good out of my life? How can I get rid of this pain and see the light again?

There were many dark moments when I felt weak and wanted to go back. I was looking for a voice to tell me to not give up, to be strong. To learn to control my emotions instead of letting them take over.

There was nothing like that, I had to figure out on my own reading many books, and talking to a lot of therapists, which tools were going to work for me and my situation, and which ones were not.

That is what this book will do; give you strategies that you can do right now to start rebuilding and healing. This book will show you the areas to work on, so you can reach your goals much faster.

I want to tell others survivors that life does get easier. That the shame and anger you feel right now is normal. Now is time to take care of you and forget about anybody else for a while.

I want to inspire other women to find the strength within them and get up, dust themselves off, total your losses and move on. **Let your journey begin.**

Chapter 1.
Do not go back

"Courage is resistance to fear, mastery of fear, not absence of fear" – Mark Twain

I knew with the first slap I should have left, and I did! But I came back. A pattern that is sadly very common in victims of domestic violence and abusive relationships.

Your ex starts to sweet talk you into coming back. "It's not going to happen again", he says. "Things got out of hand...please forgive me". So you start to doubt your judgment and start to think: "maybe he's right, I didn't give things a chance, and he has never done this before"

"Maybe I pushed him too hard?"; "Maybe it was my fault?" So you go back and try to pretend that nothing happened. I like to call this time the "honeymoon stage". Where you two find the love that united you at the beginning and things are looking good!

You're both smiling and planning for the future again. You feel happy and glad you came back, and for now, you put that incident behind you.

Then eventually very soon, it does happen again. There is another fight and things get ugly very quickly. That's when he starts to hit you and insult you, now comes a full blown abusive relationship.

Practice Leaving

You leave and try to have no contact, but the feelings of loneliness and confusion make you go back. This happens many times before you actually leave for good.

Some theorists call this "practice leaving". It's when we want to test the waters and see if we can really make it out there on our own. It's like a test we give ourselves to see if that's what really is best.

Some of us will take the kids to our parents and stay there for a few days while things calm down. Usually lying to them about the real reason you are there.

While we are out we start to miss the routine. You start to miss and remember some good times as a way to validate your own feelings of weakness and emptiness. So you go back, hoping it will be better this time.

But things do not get better, they get worse. You have to realize that you can lose your life by staying in such a relationship. You are far more precious than you think you are; never go back to someone that mistreats you either emotionally or physically.

Once you are out for good, you have to be ready to put in the work. You are going to be scared, you are going to be confused for a while, but you have to hit this head-on and hit the ground running.

Chapter 2.
It all starts with a plan

"Our goals can only be reached through a vehicle of a plan, in which we must fervently believe, and upon which we must vigorously act. There is no other route to success."

Pablo Picasso

When you are living in an abusive relationship, you rarely get to make your own decisions, let alone have any personal goals or the means to achieve them.

You are stripped of your confidence, your self-steam, and your will to fight for your dreams. You become a shell of a person that lives to cater to your partner in every way you can, at the cost of sacrificing your own life and hopes.

So once you are out on your own, it's going to feel strange that you are now your own boss. Don't waste any time, time to make some goals and carve the life you are meant to live, the life that you want.

At first, you will not know where to start, where to go, or what to do. It's like getting in your car and start driving, but you don't know where you're going.

That's why you need a plan; think of it as GPS for your life. It will help you have a course of action in case you get lost along the way; you can quickly get back on track, and keep an eye on your progress. You need directions that will help you accomplish your goals.

When you have a plan you have something to work forwards to, you have a purpose. It will give you the confidence and the strength you need to move forward.

This is the time to get excited about your future, about your hopes and dreams. This is the time to daydream. To close your eyes for a moment and imagine your life as you want it to be.

There are so many possibilities; you just have to figure out what moves you, what motivates you, what makes you happy just thinking about it?

Do you want to go back to school and finish that degree? Do you want to get that job you always wanted? Do you want to start that business you always dreamed of? The sky is really the limit.

10 Tips to help you stick with your Plan

1. **Keep a Journal**

One thing that helped me tremendously was keeping a journal. I would write down all my goals and dreams. I would make a list of the main goal, and the steps I needed to take to get there. It was a great way to jot down random thoughts, silly dreams like go to Disneyland this year. I would keep photos, mementos, and write down any goal-oriented thoughts that came to mind throughout the day. I kept it in my purse all the time. So whenever I needed a pick me up, or a sense of direction. I would open my journal and get back on track.

2. Write your main goals down

When you put your thoughts on paper, something gets ignited in your mind. It seems to activate your subconscious and your goals become impregnated in your thoughts because you have taken the physical effort to take them out of your mind, and into the paper.

This definitely can influence you greatly to take action much quicker than if you just keep them in your thoughts, where they can get lost in the thousands of ideas you have every day.

3. Focus your focus

You are not trying to change the world here; you just need to save yourself first. Start with one or two goals first, and move up from there. Pick the ones that excite you the most, the ones that you know will keep you motivated. The ones you know you will finish.

4. Devise an action plan

Once you have identified the two to three main goals you are going to focus on first, it's time to come up with an action plan. Do you already possess, or do you need to acquire new skills to achieve this goal? Who do you need to reach to? What are the steps necessary?

As you through the steps to achieve your dreams, be aware that plans may change from time to time, as you gain more insight into your own self and your abilities.

You may decide that instead of going for that dream job, you are going to go back to school and update your skills, or gain new ones!

Never be afraid to change course if life is steering you in a different direction, or your heart is telling you to go a different route.

You are now the owner of your destiny and the captain of your ship. So feel free to steer it in any direction you want, as long as you are moving forward and up.

There is no need to apologize if you're starting over, this is your life and you are in control now.

5. Visualize your goal as if they are realized

Emotions are a very powerful thing. As survivors of abuse, we know very well that emotions move us to react and feel so many things. Emotions make things real.

So when you are thinking about your end goal, put some emotion in it. If one of your goals is to get a new car, visualize yourself driving on the open road, feel the wind on your face, listen to the music on the radio. Think about the exterior color, the tires, and the dice in the mirror (if that's your thing).

Feeling your desires as if they are true has a great impact on our self-worth. Imagine yourself in that dream job, graduating with your degree, smiling and enjoying that exotic vacation. If you can feel it, you will have it.

6. Make room for your goals

If your goal is to own a home, clean up your credit, talk to a banker about your mortgage options, visit a few open houses of your dream home, start to put yourself there.

Once you start to get into the emotions of realizing your dreams, and putting yourself right in the middle of your goals, they do have a way of finding themselves realized.

It's no secret that we attract what we project, and if we project ourselves as being weak, and unsuccessful, and doubtful if we are ever going to be happy. We will attract the same mentality from others, and our own life will reflect those feelings.

Make room in your life to receive those goals, and very soon you will see yourself stop dreaming, and start living the best life you can possibly have, and more!

7. Take action daily, even in small doses
Rome was not built in a day, you've heard that a million times. But there is a very profound truth in it, slowly but surely we can all achieve great things.

Don't expect for things to happen overnight, which is why you have an action plan to guide you through all the little details, or roads, that will lead you to your destination.

Do not let a day go by that you don't take a small step in achieving your goals. No matter if it's just reading some affirmations to stay motivated, or making a phone call that will get you into a door.

We are living in a fast, fast world. The world is constantly changing and evolving, enjoy the moment. Enjoy all of your accomplishments, even if it is a small one. Giving up smoking, for example, is a great goal to have for your physical health. Celebrate those small victories and they will lead you to bigger ones.

8. **Track your progress**

If you cannot see your progress, you will not know what you have accomplished, and what else needs to be done. If you cannot see it, you cannot fix it.

Feel free to use the Goals Tracking Sheet on the opposite page as a guideline for producing your own charts and timelines. They are very helpful to show you where you are lacking, and where you are actually ahead.

You can use these to make adjustments as necessary. Use anything that will help you, an app, a piece of paper, or a notebook. Just make sure you keep it with you so you can refer to it anytime you feel lost, and to jot down what you have done already.

9. Celebrate your milestones

A great reason to track your progress is to celebrate those little successes along the way. You have worked hard; you have beaten the odds and are now making it on your own.

Large goals are made of a lot of tiny steps that as a whole; will bring you closer to living the life you were meant to live.

As you take a moment and savor your accomplishments, you will believe more than ever in your power to change your life. Now you know you can do anything.

10. Keep positive people by your side always

One of the considerations for our support system is that they need to bring positivism to your life. Constructive criticism that comes from a negative place has no place in your new life. If anybody makes you feel anything other than good about yourself and is willing to give you a break and let you grow, you have to take this person out of your life immediately.

How not to fail

The first few weeks after I left besides being confused and lost, I was very scared of what my future will bring. I did not feel strong enough to go out there in the world and face more disappointments, more hurt.

I wanted to stay in my bubble and never come out. I wanted to just cry and feel sorry for myself. Ask myself over and over again, why I had to go through something like that? When is the pain ever going to go away?

I started to think of all my failures up to that point, and how I started to follow a path that was never conducive of anything positive, in the end at least. And I realized one thing.

Whenever I set out to carve some goals, like when I decided to go back to school and get my degree after many years of being out, I always envisioned it very far in the future.

For example, I thought finishing a degree and graduating was going to take minimum three to four years. So even though I had a goal, it was kind of discouraging that it would take so long. So I decided to look at the end of a semester with passing grades, as a victory all within itself.

I would treat myself to a nice dinner at my favorite restaurant, or maybe treat myself to some new clothes or shoes. Anything that would make me happy inside I would use as a reward, and the time off from school between classes, I spent it with my family as much as I could.

Keeping that balance of celebrating my small victories, and moving forward with my goals one step at a time, was essential in rebuilding my life after an abusive relationship.

That is how you can assure you will not fail, you will not get distracted on your path, and you will stay motivated.

I wanted to prove myself to the world that I could do anything I wanted to, mostly prove it to myself that I still had it in me. Being oppressed and feeling like garbage for so long, chips away at your soul and spirit. Before you know it, you are an empty shell of what you used to be. Depression sets in and you have to make a decision. Are you going to stay down and be a doormat all your life? Or are you going to make it count and have a good life?

Make sure you are also making realistic goals. If you want to be a doctor, but you can't pass medical school, it's time to rethink and obtain a new approach. However, there are exceptions and just because there is some obstacle to your goals, does not mean you can't overcome them.

Just be aware of your limitations, and work on those weaknesses so that you can improve your chances of getting what you want. Learn as much as you can.

Perseverance and being focused on the end goal will take you far and everywhere you want to go. There is nothing better than being proud of yourself, and know that it was all you.

Use the following worksheets to work on your goals. Write on this book, or in your journal and keep making those goals. Remember, it all starts with a plan!

I recommend dedicating a Journal just for your goals. Write down how you're feeling, and how much you are progressing. Whenever you are feeling lost, refer to your journal and get yourself back on track. It's ok if it's taking time, just keep moving forward.

Write on your physical copy of the book, or reproduce this page in your own journal. Write the deadline on the last column

Example:

Goal: Get a better job in the medical field

Step 1 Look for open positions in current job   5/6/2018

Step 2 Look in job websites for openings   5/8/2018

Step 3 Do I need more training? Find out   5/10/2018

Step 4 Update Resume   5/12/2018

Step 5 Submit Resume to Job Sites/Recruiters   5/14/2018

Goal:

Step 1 _____   _____

Step 2 _____   _____

Step 3 _____   _____

Step 4 _____   _____

Goal:

Step 1 _____ _____

Step 2 _____ _____

Step 3 _____ _____

Step 4 _____ _____

Goal:

Step 1 _____ _____

Step 2 _____ _____

Step 3 _____ _____

Step 4 _____ _____

Goal:

Step 1 _____ _____

Step 2 _____ _____

Step 3 _____ _____

Step 4 _____ _____

Goal:

Step 1 _____ _____

Step 2 _____ _____

Step 3 _____ _____

Step 4 _____ _____

Chapter 3.
How to stay safe

The days following my scape were so nerve-wracking; every single noise would make me jump and scream. I was scared of the wind, any noise, or anyone I didn't see coming. I was so scared he would drag me into his car, take me to some remote location and kill me.

The police were just taking reports and not doing anything else, just waiting for him to show up and hurt me I guess. I was pregnant; I couldn't drive or defend myself physically. If he grabbed me on the street, I thought, it could be bad.

When I finally got the restraining order I was somewhat relieved. I understood that it was a strong deterrent to keep him away, but will it really? I wasn't sure. So I spent the next few days looking out the window and going out as little as possible. I was really scared.

Regain control

- **Move**

Your safety is so much more important than any place. Leaving our familiar surroundings, neighbors, schools, work, etc. can be very overwhelming and extremely scary. But it can also be exactly what you need, a fresh start, and new surroundings.

- **Keep it in the Down Low (DL)**

Don't stop there. Change your number, email address, and go by a different name in your social media accounts. Make yourself as less visible as possible. You don't want to taunt your abuser into finding you and hurting you by disclosing your location anywhere on the internet.

You may think is harmless to post a picture of your new relationship with your kids happy and smiling, but an ex who may be monitoring your activity, may not react so harmless. Keep your social media closed tight, and if possible, just ignore it all together. You don't have to be sharing your life for others to see, focus on growing real relationships where physical contact is what counts.

- **Alert your Support System**

Surround yourself with people that will look out for you and protect you. Some may not believe the kind of danger that you are in, and innocently (or not) disclose your location to your abuser. Be careful who you trust, and keep your circle small.

If you fear that your children may be in danger of kidnapping, or anything that can put them in harm's way, notify your local police and file a report.

Inform their teachers and school administrators of your situation. Tell them that your ex cannot pick up the kids from school under any circumstance. If they are not cooperative, seek help from the police.

- **Talk to your Kids**

If your kids are old enough, talk to them. Try to keep the conversation light, and instead of rambling and sugar coating the situation, let them ask questions. Let it flow naturally, and assure them they haven't done anything wrong.

As a parent, you will know when it's time to seek professional help, and I encourage you to do so anyway. There is only so much we can do as parents, getting a therapist or a psychologist can help you and your children cope and heal.

- **If you must go into hiding**

The most dangerous time after you leave an abusive relationship is right after you leave. He is going to look for you, beg you to come back, promise you that things are going to change, that things will be fine. But they never will be, you cannot trust anyone at this point, and you must also protect yourself.

Just because the danger is not staring at you, doesn't mean is not near. You must stay alert at all times, and be aware of anything out of the ordinary around you. Always be on the lookout for any car circling your block, anonymous calls to your phone, or anyone following you home from work or school.

Always be alert, and don't ever be afraid to call the police if you feel you are in danger. Be proactive.

- **If you need a restraining order**

Once you have moved out and are on your own. You must contact authorities and file a police report any time there is an altercation. You want to have those complaints on file in case you need to file a restraining order or obtain any protection from the police.

I had a really bad experience with the police. Some didn't believe me when I told them my boyfriend was hitting me. I just couldn't believe that they would look at me, a pregnant woman in tears, turn themselves around and completely dismiss me.

It wasn't until things got really bad, and he started to follow me everywhere I went. Sometimes he would pull up next to me in his car, scream at me to pull over and talk to him. He would come around my mother's house when my car was there, knocking on the door nonstop, trying to force himself inside the house to talk to me.

I had no choice than to protect myself and my child. I had to get a restraining order. The process varies from state to state, so your best bet is to call your local office where they handle these types of things. A simple Google search will do.

Follow these tips to file your restraining order:

1. Gather all if any evidence you have on what's been happening. Any text messages, emails, phone calls, voicemails, pictures of bruises and lesions, and witness accounts. You have to prove to the court that you are being harassed, and definitely in danger, so having hard proof this will help you greatly.

2. If you get a court date, hire a lawyer. If you cannot afford one, there is a legal aid program in every state where you can procure free legal representation.

3. During court, the judge will scrutinize you and judge you harshly. There are a lot of fraudulent claims for restraining orders, so the judge will want to make sure yours is genuine.

4. As survivors of domestic abuse, we want to appear tough and show that we can stand up for ourselves. However, your court date is not the day for that. The best advice I got from my lawyer was that we have to show ourselves like the victims that we are (even though we are victims no more once we are out).

5. When you show up for court dress modestly, watch your voice volume and tone. It's easy to get angry and start shouting at your abuser about how you feel, but

the judge will not see it your way. Stay humble, speak clearly and tell your story as eloquent as you can. It's ok to get emotional and shed a few tears, you have been through a lot, just leave your anger out of court.

6. After you are awarded your order, make copies of the official paper and keep the original with you at all times. I usually keep it in my glove compartment in my car. The copies are to be distributed to anyone that needs to come in contact with you or your children. Your children's school administrator, your job, if you have security where you live they need a copy.

Having a support system was crucial during this time. I found refuge in my family and in my new baby. I was so full of love for my little one, so much hope, that thinking negatively became less and less frequent.

Some Legal resources you may find helpful. First, do a search in your area to see what legal assistance you have available close by. Make sure you are safe when contacting anyone.

American Bar Association Commission on Domestic Violence
1-202-662-1000   www.abanet.org/domviol

Battered Women's Justice Project
1-800-903-0111   www.bwjp.org

The National Domestic Violence Hotline
1-800-799-7233 (SAFE)   www.ndvh.org

Chapter 4.
You can't do this alone

One of the hardest things I ever had to do was come clean to my family and friends about what was happening to me. I felt an overwhelming mix of feelings. I felt like a failure, ashamed, and disappointment in myself. I didn't want anyone to know what I was going through, so I hid what was going on for a long time.

I always gave the impression of being this strong woman who didn't take crap from anyone, who was making her own way in the world, who could do anything on her own. Instead, I had become weak, dependent, defeated. What was left was a vague representation of the strong woman I used to be.

When I decided to leave, I knew that the first step was to come clean to my family and close friends. It was not going to be easy, probably one of the hardest and most painful things I've ever had to do. Admit that I had been living practically in hell, abused, beaten, and left with a very shattered soul.

One thing that certainly pushed me over the edge and convinced me to tell my family what was happening, was something my mother in law told me, and surprisingly she made a lot of sense to me. In essence, she said, "your family will always be there for you, no matter what.

Whether you are guilty or not, they will take your side and protect you. Go to them, don't be ashamed you did nothing wrong."

That statement really resonated with me. People were suspecting and knew something was wrong, but I think we're afraid to ask me and find out the truth.

When I finally told them, it was a huge relief on my part, and I was able to talk about what happens much easier after that. Getting their help in letting me in so I can get myself together, played a very vital role in me getting the space I needed to get away, regroup, refocus, and move on with my life.

You cannot do this alone. If you don't have a place to go, you are going to need somebody to help you get out. You're going to need somebody to lean on for the moment.

You have to put your shame aside and think about you for a second. Because you matter; you deserve to be free. If you have kids, you really don't need any other reason. They deserve the best, and you can give it to them. But you have to be free first.

One of the textbook classic tactics of a narcissist is the fact that they want you all for themselves. They lose control over you if you get close to anybody other than them. They will do anything to smear your reputation so that nobody will want anything to do with you.

I really recommend you find somebody you can trust to help you. The days after you leave your abuser can be the most dangerous. That's when feelings are really fresh and you will feel very confused. Having somebody to talk to, to find comfort in, or just to lend you a couch to crash while you figure it out, can make all the difference in whether you go back to hell, or make it on your own.

How to find your support team

1. Start by making a list of all the people in your life you think will understand what you're going through, and who will help you in your transition.

2. Go through your list again, prioritize who you are going to call first, and have a conversation with them about your situation.

3. You have to be able to trust them, or they can actually hurt you more. They can warn your abuser about your plans. Avoid anyone in his family; no matter how you close you think you are to them. In the end, family sticks with family.

4. Never leave a toxic relationship to start a new one. If anyone will bring negativity into your life, stay away from them. Yes, including family.

5. Be careful who you tell your story. Not everyone will sympathize, and some may even judge you for it. Protect yourself from negativity by never leading with your past.

6. Only contact ex-lovers if you know you can trust them as friends. Be careful of being used when you are at your most vulnerable.

7. Be safe. If you fear for your safety and don't have access to a cell phone of your own, use somebody

else's phone, friends or a family member you can trust. If you can, call one person and have them contact the other people you need to get in touch with. Be very careful about this.

8. Do not overstay your welcome.
   Communicate to the people that are helping you with your plans and be very clear. Letting them know what you actually plan to do, and how you are going to do it, will assure them that you are on your way to being on your own.

You will not start to feel like yourself again until you are in your own space. Where you are free to make your own rules, your own routine, and give yourself and your family some stability.

It's ok to dream big, write them down, and visualize yourself with that degree, that dream job, that vacation you always wanted, that new car. Life is there for the taking, so it might as well be you.

Chapter 5.
How to beat your number one enemy

Have you ever cried so hard you can't make a sound? Have you ever cried so deeply that your chest feels like a knife is going through it? I felt my heart breaking in a million pieces. I tried to find comfort by thinking about holding my baby. But I would also start to remember the fights, the humiliations in public, the punches in the middle of the night, kicking me until I fell to the floor.

All of the sudden this hot and heavy rage consumes me. I start screaming to the top of my lungs, AAAAAAAHHHHHHHH……AAAAAHHHHHHHH, I can't stop screaming with heavy tears running down my eyes. I start to punch the walls, kick the furniture, throw picture frames around and glass is breaking everywhere. I am in full rage mode being seven months pregnant. I felt so out of control, it was almost uncontrollable.

I wanted to break stuff, I wanted to break myself. I would grab my hair and try to pull it out, I felt out of control. I would throw myself on the floor to cry, to punch the ground, to punch the walls; it was really heartbreaking to have those feelings.

Your number one enemy in this period of recovery, and in any other period of your life, is **anger**.
I was so angry at everything, myself mostly. I beat myself up pretty good. I would lie in bed and just cry myself to

sleep. Then the next day I would feel horrible, abandoned, impotent, and embarrassed. I felt so stupid for letting myself get into such a chaotic situation.

What happened to me? I was supposed to be smart and make all the right decisions, and I clearly made a horrible choice. The embarrassment of carrying a child out of wedlock from a man who wants to hurt me? Sometimes it was too much to think about so it would trigger those feelings of anger and rage. It was almost unbearable for my mind to handle.

At that moment I understood why some people go crazy and lose their minds. Why they do unbelievable things out of rage and anger. I tried to calm myself by thinking that I was safe, he couldn't get to me at least for now. I also had my new baby to think about.

This is when you have to pause, thank God for what you do have, and pray for the strength you need to start feeling better.

I open my journal and look up a list I made of all the wonderful things happening for me right now (you should do one too!). I see a picture of my baby, my future college degree, and that beautiful home I will soon own.

Strategies to overcome this enemy

- **Just Breathe**

It is not easy at first. Trying to sit still and concentrate on your breathing can be pretty hard, but with practice and dedication, you will learn to substitute negative thoughts for positive ones. Your life will start reflecting your new positive attitude, and you will be able to attract the same into your life.

Just close your eyes, breathe, and feel the love all over you. Feel loved and project that love onto yourself. All of the sudden I was smiling, I was relaxed, I was feeling charged up and ready, I was ready for my life to begin.

So from that point on, I made a constant effort to keep my emotions under control. Focusing on my future and the work I needed to make right now to make it happen kept me pretty busy. There were days better than others, and sometimes I had to take a moment and just be and have a cry, I did feel sad sometimes.

So the next time I felt the anger creeping in and taking over, I just closed my eyes and breathe, trying to concentrate on my breathing and letting the thoughts of anger just flow through me. I just watched them come and leave. I focused on my thoughts for the future and how I envision my life to be.

But if I was going to make it out, I had to find a way to bring myself back.
So little by little, and breath by breath, I did. And you can too, just breathe.

Don't hold to anger, hurt or pain. They steal your energy and keep you from love." — **Leo Buscaglia**

- **Stop Stewing**

During the first few days and weeks after I left him, there were some nights when I couldn't sleep. I would go over in my mind the events that led me to leave: the night he tackled me to the floor from a chair, the black eyes and the bruises.

At the same time, I would think of the good times. About how we met, how smitten and happy we were with each other and the plans we had. I was just a ball of emotions. I was missing him, I hated him. I was wishing he would disappear, I was wishing I never met him.

It wasn't until I realized what I was doing, I was stewing and stewing those memories based on lies. Just like when you simmer a soup for hours and hours to get that rich flavor, we hope the same will happen with our feelings and thoughts of the past.

By stewing the past you are looking for ways to justify abuse, mistreatment, and physical violence all in the name of love. You are looking for an easy way out; you are looking for an excuse to go back.

One day I just said "STOP! STOP! STOP! "I have to stop going over in my head what I could have done differently, what I should have said and the hell I was living. I had to stop myself from getting in my own way.

Ove the next few days, I just tried really hard to stay busy. As long as I was being productive and kept it moving, I was fine. Day by day my new life was getting filled with new routines, new things to do, new worries, and sometimes new problems.

I can't remember how long after this happened, but one day I just woke up and it was all gone, well most of it. The anger, the anguish, the self-doubt, the shame, the embarrassment, the fear, all these confused feelings of being in limbo, were suddenly less present.

I woke up energized, ready to tackle my new life, ready to be a mom. My anxiety turned out to be about me and my new future. I just couldn't wait to move on and create new memories.

It felt so good to realize that things finally were looking up for me. I had a different outlook on life, and it was all sinking in finally. I was going to be okay.

"Follow your bliss and the universe will open doors where there were only walls"

Joseph Campbell

"Anger, resentment, and jealousy don't change the heart of others-- it only changes yours."
Shannon L. Alder

- **Do Something Physical**

If you wanted to get in shape, well this is the time! Running, cycling, yoga, weights, whatever you fancy to do at the gym or outside, being physical is a healthy way to release stress. Even if it's just a walk around the block, use this time to meditate, to breath, to enjoy nature. In time your mind and body will thank you.

- **Do something nice**

Get takeout from your favorite restaurant, buy the bottle of wine and soak in the tub. Pamper yourself a little, even if it's just taking a much-needed nap. Feeling good and happy inside will make you less prone to react to any situation that will prompt you to be angry.

Sometimes, also doing something nice for somebody else we love can bring a great sense of happiness. Volunteering in a senior home or a hospital, can bring life into focus and make you appreciate your life, even more, making you less angry.

- **Seek help if you need it**

If life becomes too overwhelming and the feelings of anger are taking over your life, please never be afraid to seek help from a therapist.

One of the best decisions of my life was to speak with a psychologist. Sometimes having somebody to just listen and give you some tools to deal with your anger in a constructive way, can be of great help and will help you heal much faster.

Look for a therapist that specializes in victims of violence and/or sexual abuse. Finding a good therapist can be daunting, and it will probably take a few tries before you find the right one for you. Don't be afraid to walk away from a session if it's not helping at all.

Give therapy a chance, and you may be surprised at the results. Ultimately you will have to put in the work, but being guided by a professional who wants to see you succeed, can make all the difference.

Don't forget to do a google search in your own hometown to see what you have available in your area.

Affirmations:

- I am in control
- I remain calm even when under intense stress
- I always speak my mind rather than let frustrations build up
- I am able to calm myself down and detach from anger
- I am gaining more and more control over my emotions
- I owe it to myself to manage my anger

National Suicide Prevention Lifeline (1-800-273-8255).
Trained crisis workers are available to talk 24 hours a day, 7 days a week.
Calls are confidential and toll-free.

Substance Abuse and Mental Health Services Administration (SAMHSA)
Treatment Referral Helpline at 1-800-662-HELP (4357)
Find a health care provider or treatment locator

To find facilities where you pay according to your income, go to https://www.hrsa.gov/

You can also go to the website of your state or county government and search for the health services department.

To learn more about mental health, visit https://www.mentalhealth.gov/

Chapter 6.
Get your finances in order

Making money while under the watch of an abuser can be very challenging. They want to be involved in everything you do, especially when it comes to money. This is how they gain the most control over you. If you have no money, you can't do anything, you can't run.

You need to regain control over this aspect of your life, and you need to get your finances in order.

Take inventory
What do you have to your name? A car, a Real State property, a bank account with some savings? A piggy bank? Anything of value that you can sell to make money if you need to, should be accounted for.

If you have income or savings
If you are currently working, start to save money by putting aside any money you have left after paying the bills. Forget about the fancy coffee, the mani, and pedi. During this period all luxuries must be put on hold. You need to start focusing on establishing a money fund for your future.

Setup a budget based on what you will need to survive if you lose your job today. You need to save enough money to survive without an income for at least six months.

Nine ways to get cash if you have no income or savings

If you are unemployed, you need to start looking for a job as soon as possible. It's time to stand on your own two feet and get back out there.

Polish that resume and update it, register on job boards and start practicing interviewing. There are tons of resources online, find one that works for you.

1. **Search for jobs in your area**

If you are able to use the internet, do a google search for "jobs near me" This will bring up jobs advertised in your area, you will be surprised how many openings you can find.
Jobs in retail stores, local small companies and business are going to be easier to get. When you apply for these jobs, make sure the schedule is going to work for you. If you need to get the kids to and from school, make sure your new job will allow you to do that, or find adequate after school care so you can work.

This is where having a support system of one or more people will really help. You need to make money for your future, and you need to work to get it. Your support group should be able to lend you a hand with your children if you need to be at work.

2. Job Apps and Websites

Sites like TaskRabbit, Craigslist and even Facebook Marketplace are flooded with requests from local neighbors looking for help for a variety of tasks. Some are just for a day or longer. Everything from tutoring to yard work to house painting can be found online. Post an ad or register to look for these jobs, and you can have cash on your hands today.

3. Welcome to the "Share Economy".

Companies like Uber, Airbnb, Lyft, and others, are empowering people like you and me to be our own boss and work our own hours. My brother drives for Lyft, and he makes a decent amount of income just working part-time.

4. Housekeeper

A simple google search in your area for cleaning companies, either for residential or commercial spaces, should yield a fair amount of businesses for you to get hired immediately. If you have a few references and the physical ability, cleaning houses and offices is a good way to get some needed cash fast. Some pay daily. Why not start your own housekeeping business?

5. Walk dogs, Pet Sitting

Dog owners are very passionate about their "little children" as they like to call them. Many of them are forced to leave them alone in the house for many hours while they go to work. They would love someone they trust to go into their house and walk their dog outside so they are happy. They will pay you extra to fill their bowl with food, administer medications, or maybe just to hang out with their pet while they are at work.

6. Babysit

Parents are everywhere that need someone they can trust to watch their kids for a while. Adults need adult time sometimes, and that's when you come in. Spread the word to your friends and family that you are available to babysit, for a modest fee. However, don't be afraid to ask the going rate, after all, you are taking a huge responsibility. Sign up for any of these jobs and more online, fill up your profile with as much information as needed, and once you become available, you will be on your way to an income stream.

7. Virtual Assistant

Sign up on sites like Upwork and Fiverr for short term contracts and tasks. You can set your own rates, and pick the jobs you want to work on. You would be doing things like internet research, audio transcribing, ad posting, and other related tasks.

8. Sell Something

Are you still holding on to that old dress that you wore once ten years ago? Do you have jewelry that is attached to a painful memory? Do your kids have too many toys that they have outgrown and are taking over your life? Sell all that stuff! You'd be surprised at what people buy these days.

So go ahead and look around, you have things you can get rid of, things that are holding you back. Heavy things like exercise machines, furniture, and big bulky toys your kids probably don't use anymore sell very well.

When you finish gathering what you want to sell, there are many ways you get cash:

- eBay (Sell anything! Great for easy to ship items and collectibles)
- Offer Up, Let Go (phone app)
- Poshmark (clothing and shoes selling App)
- Craigslist (Always meet at a police station)
- Facebook local marketplace
- Yard Sale
- Pawn Shops (jewelry, electronics)

Things that sell well:

- Electronics, old classics, and newer models
- Video Games
- Bicycles, Exercise Machines

- Toys
- Collectibles, antiques (Unique and old)
- Baby items (Crib, stroller, car seat, etc.)
- Furniture (In good condition, antique)
- Gold and Silver Jewelry

9. **Get a Loan**

You are going to need money to help get yourself together. You are going to need to get a new place, money to put the kids in daycare, in school, buy groceries, etc. Especially if you know your "soon to be ex" is not going to help you.

If you are lucky to have someone willing to invest in you and your future by giving you a loan, make sure you share your plan with them. Let them know that you are on your way to get back on track, and you will pay them as soon as possible.

I know how hard it is to find somebody who will loan you money when you are not working; this is why getting a support system consisting of people you can count on is important. Remember, you will never know unless you ask, and pride needs to be put aside for now.

How to create a budget and stick to it

It is so important to create a budget and stick to it as much as possible. It is important to be aware of how much you are spending, versus how much you are making. Make adjustments to either expenses or income when necessary is a part of staying on track with your finances, and not overspend.

Having a budget will help you be prepared for the unforeseeable expenses, and there will be many. Flat tires, medical bills, vacations, etc. Now that you are on your own, you are going to need to have a nest egg, a cushion.

To help you get started in creating a budget, follow the following tips:

1. If there any overages in your budget, you have money left over after you cover all your basic expenses. Open a savings account and transfer 90 percent of that amount every month.

2. Give yourself an allowance
   maybe weekly or monthly treat yourself to a little cash. Buy a nice lunch at work or get your hair done. Great way to stay motivated, love yourself too.

3. Plan meals and shop ahead
   nothing eats at your budget like eating out. Plus, you will consume many unnecessary calories and fat that will make you and your family gain weight and face health problems. Be good to you and your wallet, and plan your meals ahead of time.

4. Set Goals
   If you want to buy that new car, or finally buy your first home or pay off your current one. Make a goal out of

it, when you define it and put in front of you, you are more likely to succeed.

5. Build an emergency fund
   Six months of expenses in a savings account earning interest.

6. Involve the entire family
   when you involve your family in your budget and saving money, they can all learn valuable lessons and help you stay on track. My daughter helps me clip coupons and look for sales!

7. Keep a journal of everything you buy for one week
   that daily $1.50 cup of coffee may not seem like much, but multiplied times 20 times a month? That's $30 a month, that's $360 a year!

8. Suppress the need to cheat on your budget
   We all have those urges, but sticking to your guns will not only make you feel proud of yourself, but it will also help you accomplish your goals!

Learning how to budget your finances is a very good skill to transfer to your kids. You will be giving them real-life skills that they can take with them into adulthood, and help them be responsible with money.

One of the main reasons women stay with their abuser is because of finances, they have no money to go anywhere. Make sure you are always able to support yourself, and have cash available for any unexpected expenses.

Having something to fall back can bring on major confidence, and will make things easier should you need to change your situation again in the future. Always have a plan.

Use the following Budget Sheet as a guide to help you get started in creating your budget. Feel free to modify it to fit your needs.

Sample Budget Sheet

Income: _____

Expenses:
Mortgage/Rent: _____

Utilities: _____

Credit Cards: _____

Insurance: _____

Car Payments: _____

Cell Phone: _____

Groceries: _____

Gasoline: _____

Child Care: _____

Misc.: _____

Total Expenses: $_____

(-)Total Income: $_____

Difference or Over: $_____

Chapter 7.
How to get back on your feet, fast

What a beautiful thing it is, to be able to stand tall and say, "I felt apart, and I survived."
-The new you

Put yourself first

One of the many traits that we women possess is the need to fix everything around us, including people. That has to stop today! You have no control over anyone's actions. The only thing you can control is you, and what you do in your own life.

You have to stop being a doormat; you have to stop living for others, what about you? Who helps you? Who cares about you? In the end, you have to do what's best for you.

Be selfish, is ok! Go and get that massage, go to the beach, go to the gym, take care of yourself first. Learn how to say no to people, trust me they will understand. For years I put other's needs first before mine, I helped others even when I needed the help first. Once I saw myself alone with a baby, with no one around to help me, I realized I had to start living for me.

When you take care of your needs first and start saying no to every situation you get pulled in, will condition your friends and family to know that you are not always available. That you too have responsibilities and things you need to get done. It is not all about them anymore.

Being selfish does not mean you don't care about others. It just means that you are taking care of yourself first, and then others.

Especially when you are in a vulnerable state, make sure that your emotional and physical needs are met. Only then you can turn around and take care of somebody else.

If you have children, this is a very important step. You need to take the time to recover emotionally, and being selfish with yourself at this time is perfectly fine.

You need time to become more secure in yourself and your own abilities, give yourself that break and focus on your life.

Love you for you

One of the things that helped me the most in the aftermath was falling in love with me again.
I started to appreciate little things about myself like my laugh, my new positive attitude towards life, my compassion for others, and even my sense of humor! I was laughing again!

It was not an overnight process at all. At first, it hurt to laugh, it hurt to feel good because it's been so bad for so long. But I just couldn't let myself be discouraged, and little by little, day by day, I felt more and more comfortable in my own skin.

After much meditation and thinking about why I let myself into such an abusive and violent situation, I realized that it was my longing for acceptance and love that drove me into it.

As a child, I was often put to the side, not given too much importance. I was often compared to my other siblings, "why can't you be more like your sister" type of thing.

This created a sense of not belonging anywhere. I longed so much to be accepted by my mother and father, friends, anyone, that I became a doormat for anyone that would give me any type of attention. And that feeling grew with me into adulthood and men.

Even if the guy was a known liar, even if I knew for sure that he was with me just for the physical part, I still stayed. Even as fake and as superficial as his attention was, I wanted it. It made me feel like I mattered to someone and that got me into a situation where I was taken advantage of.

I wanted love from everyone so bad, that I forgot to love myself. I forgot how much I mattered and how much I was worth. I forgot that I deserved to be cherished and respected, loved and understood.

Instead, I gave my all of myself in exchange for a little love, a little attention. What was left was a desolated place where I only found solace, depression, and sadness. I was sinking into a big dark hole that was becoming my life.

Luckily somehow one day I just woke up. That day when I found myself on the floor after being punched in the face by my baby's father, drowning in my tears, feeling the most horrible pain in my heart. I realized that I had to get myself out. I needed to feel like myself again.

Stop the negativity

Stop the negative thoughts about yourself. What happened to you was not your fault, you are not stupid, or naïve or dumb. The fact that domestic abuse is an issue that is not talked about much makes us feel isolated, and make us feel like we are the only one going through something like this.

However, domestic violence happens every day to millions of people; you are a very lucky person to be reading this. That means you made it out! Be proud of that! Stop beating yourself up and keep moving forward towards your goals.

Avoid perfectionism

You are human; you are going to make mistakes. It is how we deal with them that makes us great, or not. If you keep falling in the same vicious cycle you are not learning, you are not growing.

Stop trying to achieve the impossible, know your limits and abilities. Most importantly, be ok with them. You don't have to be a doctor or a lawyer, just be the best YOU that you can be, and be the best at it. That goes for anything you try to accomplish.

Also remember, you are not a finished product. You will continue to learn, continue to grow. You will make more mistakes (hopefully not the same ones), but you will make some more. It's what makes you human. Accepting them and learning from them is what makes us stronger every day.

Accept yourself for who you are, with all your flaws and talents. Being a perfectionist will make you think that you're never good enough, stop that! That is self-defeating and you're demoralizing yourself.

It's all about setting realistic goals so you don't set yourself up for failure. Become aware of your potential by examining things you are good at, instead of trying to be somebody you are not.

Stay strong

Once you are out of an abusive relationship, you are forced to face the truth of what happened. If you have been pretending to the outside world for so long that everything is ok, now is the moment when you are confronted and forced to deal with your truth.

The trick is to not let it become you, instead, meditate on what circumstances led to that relationship becoming toxic. In the future, learn to look for red flags on people that might become abusive later on.

This is a very confusing time. You have made so many changes, and it can be very overwhelming. However, you have to remind yourself that you are strong, that you left for a reason.

The first few nights on my own, he would not leave me alone. The phone calls, the texts were nonstop. However, I stood up for myself and had become convinced that there was no way back. This is where I take control of my life.

I was not going back this time. I registered back into college, I was about to start taking online classes. I was going to my doctor's appointments to make sure the baby was coming okay.

I was making plans for the future and I was excited. I was not going to let anything or anyone derail me from making my dreams come true.

As time went on, I began to experience a rollercoaster of emotions that went from being happy to be angry and to feel sad.

I had to find strength from way deep within me to keep me safe. I meditated, I prayed, I talked to my baby. I was determined that the chaos going around me was not going to affect my decision to take control again.

Give time a chance

The first few months alone with my daughter were very rough. I was sleep deprived, I could not eat, and I was running out of money. I was feeling stressed all the time and very anxious as to how I was going to survive on my own with a brand new child.

Sometimes the anger would creep in. Just when I couldn't be more tired, I would sink back into a depression that quickly would turn into rage. I felt so angry at myself, at my situation. I felt so alone and hurt.

Sometimes I doubted that I was going to stay away this time, I felt so tempted to fall back into the familiar, which by now I have realized it was actually hell.

It has been two months and I was still miserable. The days were passing by so quickly, but my hurt was standing still chipping away at me every day. Until one day, must have been in the third month being free, when I suddenly felt lighter, less sad. I didn't have the uncontrollable need to cry and scream and break stuff. I was surprisingly calm.

And that's when I realized, I need to let time do its magic and help me heal. Letting the feelings come and go, and just learning to not react to every painful memory whenever I was triggered was critical to my recovery.

Taking it day by day and continuing meditating, I began to feel so much stronger than before. I found myself laughing every now and then; I began to enjoy life for the first time in a very long time.

As I looked into the horizon depicting a beautiful red sunset, I learned that a mistake does not define you. It also does not necessarily reflect who you are at the core.

In time, the wound you think will never close suddenly feels less painful. Every morning I felt a little stronger, a little more empowered to get over the hurt and pain. I started to feel like myself again, and it was great!

I was making new friends, and was finally talking about other things other than myself. I was smiling again. I finally started to feel happy again. It was the most incredible feeling.

It felt great to be able to be optimistic about the future. I was even contemplating dating! That's when I knew I was on the right path. I was on my way to finally being free.

> *"The most courageous act is still to think for yourself. Aloud."*
> — _Coco Chanel_

Go easy on yourself

As the days turned into weeks, I started to notice that my mind was becoming clearer and clearer. I could focus on my goals and start making the necessary steps to achieve them.

And then you have your bad days, those little setbacks that can be triggered by stablishing contact or reliving a memory. The anger will come back and the self-imposed blame for allowing such a horrible person ruin your life. For a while I was embarrassed, I was ashamed. I didn't want to talk to anyone.

I was such a strong person. I always stood on my own two feet; I always stood up for myself. Now I was a shred of that, I was on the floor.

A friend of mine came up to me and said, "Are you ok?", "Yes, I am ok". It was a lie and he knew it. You could read it on my face a mile away that there was a dark cloud storming on me. "It's ok if you're not, you have been through a very traumatic experience, if you're not ok, just go easy on yourself."

And just like that, I realized that yes, I was grieving, I was sad, I was lonely, I was going crazy a little bit. And that was OK! I need to do all of that, let it all out, let it go through me and away from me.

Once I was able to externalize my feelings and what they really were doing to me, turning me into this sad and depressed existence, I decided to forgive myself and just move on.

I was tired to constantly try to understand why I got myself into such an abusive relationship. Why I let these people destroy my life so bad that it basically left it in shambles?

I was so exhausted of blaming myself, blaming my family, blaming him, and then myself again. I was tired of blaming the circumstances, blaming my heart and my judgement.

I had to come to a place of understanding, of self-compassion. I just had to let go and stop beating myself up. It was just not getting me anywhere, actually was making things worse.

After much meditation I just came to the conclusion that the path to happiness is not going to be always a straight one. I will probably make more mistakes and set myself back a little bit. I just had to keep moving forward through the difficulties.

I had to remember that every mistake or triumph was part of my journey. Ever mishap, every move was a step in the right direction as long as it was moving towards my goals.

Getting back up was not easy at first, but it did get easier with time. Soon enough I started to feel like me again. Little by little I began to feel hopeful and my attitude changed as well. I was ready for anything.

I made a promise that I will never let anyone else control and take over my life again. Never again let anyone shame me or humiliate me to keep me under control. And never ever let anyone put their hands on me.

There were days that were very good, and some that were not so good. I would smile, get things done, enjoy my daughter, enjoy being free. And then there were dark days.

However, as time went on, those darker days turned into light gray, then those became fewer and fewer.

I always heard people say, "time heals all wounds", and now I am a firm believer in that statement. In time, your mind will substitute your feelings with whatever is happening at the moment, and those bad memories will fade. They won't disappear, but they will become less painful.

Take the time to completely heal from an abusive relationship, especially an emotional one where you lost yourself. It's easy to get swept into a romance early on when we are vulnerable and raw. Take your time.

Work on getting strong and confident. Understand how you got into your past situation, so you can be aware of the red flags in any new relationship.

Go easy on yourself, you have gone through enough.

Affirmations

Read these when you are feeling down or lost.

I deserve to be happy.

I forgive myself and set myself free.

I love and accept myself.

My mistakes do not define me.

I can always turn around and start again

I believe in me - I am willing to let go

I welcome good things in my life

I am loved - I am beautiful - I am at peace

The past is the past - Day by day

I am willing to ask for help if I need it

I will listen to my intuition more and more

I grab life by the neck, and make it go my way

Chapter 8.
Why being alone is good for you now

So you have made it out safe and are now wondering, so now what? How do I begin? Why do I feel so alone? For those in long-term relationships, there were so many years of doing the same thing, fighting the same fights, and feeling miserable day after day, that when you find yourself in a safe place away from all of that, you don't know what to do with yourself.

The loneliness creeps in and you start to freak out. Can I do this by myself? How am I going to support my children? Would I ever be safe? Should I go back? Did I try to fix things?

Being alone is scary, it's liberating, is empowering. It's finally being able to make your own decisions. You are going to be scared but you have to keep moving forward. Do not let fear get in the way of becoming your true self.

Remember always why you left, all the misery and hell because this is the time when you are more likely to go back to your abuser. Stay strong and follow these simple tips to stay on track and strong.

Make a promise to yourself:
I deserve to be happy

You owe it to yourself to never let anyone else steal your happiness. You do not deserve to be mistreated, abused, or lied to. You deserve someone that puts your happiness at the top of their priorities, never forget that.

Never settle for less

Take a moment to meditate on the good that lives in you. Take a moment to realize that as a survivor and a fighter, you deserve the life you want to live: happy and free.

Never again settle for somebody who lessens your way of life. Never again let anyone dull your spark, take away your smile. If they don't make you happy, get rid of them, fast. Whoever they are, it doesn't matter.

Think about this before anything new

Being single and not in a relationship, is a great time to reflect on what you want out of a partner in your future. What is going to make you happy? How can you avoid another abusive relationship? Sometimes our need to fix people, to solve their problems, to fit in, to belong in a group, makes us susceptible to this kind of treatment.

Now that you are alone, become aware of this and meditate on it. Think about it and understand it so that you can spot it in your future relationships. You have to make a promise to yourself that no one is going to mistreat you again, period. The only way to avoid that is to make sure your standards are not sacrificed.

If you need to make a list go ahead, and call it your "non-negotiables", what you absolutely need from a partner before anything gets serious.

You can put things like 1. Have a good job/career. 2. Live alone 3. No kids 4. Non-Smoker 5. Educated

If you have those things clear up front, you are less likely to settle for somebody who is going to lessen your quality of life.

Join a support group

Learning about other people's stories of abuse, and realizing how much in common they have with your own situation, will make you realize that you are not alone in this. Nor you are the only one in the world suffering this way.

When you communicate with others who have gone through a similar or same situation, you can receive extremely helpful insight into your life. You can also receive invaluable support from other survivors, who will make you appreciate the fact that you got out and are now working towards being happy and free.

Support groups are nowadays easy to find and join. Before social media and the Internet, to join a support group you would have to drive someplace and stand in front of a group of strangers, tell them your darkest and painful secrets. It was intimidating and very scary to expose yourself like that. But now, you can join support groups using social media outlets like Facebook and Instagram, and connect with people who like you, have gone through abusive relationships of many kinds.

These groups are great because you can seek support by just using an app on your phone; anywhere you have an internet connection and some privacy.

Whether you use Facebook, Reddit, and other independent websites and apps, you can find people from all over the world who are willing to share their stories and help others with lessons learned.

Some groups will allow you to post anonymously if you need to. You can also create a profile and actually make real connections with real people who want to help you.

Head over to Facebook for example, and just with a simple search, you can find support groups catering to survivors of domestic abuse, and many other topics related to that.

In any of those groups, you will find hundreds of members willing to give you feedback on your situation, or help you find some assistance if you are in urgent need.

Consider joining a support group today and start the healing process. It really helps to hear from others that there is another way; you don't have to stay in a situation that is not safe. There is a way out if you really want it.

Make sure your phone or computer is safe to use, and you know how to erase your history. Stay safe!

Chapter 9.
Control this emotion so you can finally move on

"Our doubts are traitors, and make us lose the good we oft might win, by fearing to attempt."
William Shakespeare

The day after I was out, when I was finally free, my mind was a complete rollercoaster of emotions. I felt so afraid and so lost. How can I make it out there on my own? Am I strong enough?

I thought about going back, which is the easy way out. Maybe it was not so bad, I thought. "Maybe if I put a little more effort into standing up for myself, maybe he will listen and stop being so rough?"

This emotion that you need to keep under control is **self-doubt**.

Going back and forth in my mind whether I should stay away or go back gave me great anxiety. Trying to make excuses for his behavior to justify going back, but also thinking of the abuse almost drove me completely crazy!

There will be days when you will question everything. You will start to feel very uncertain and confused about what your future looks like. You'll feel totally incapable of handling what is happening in your life at the moment, you lack the confidence to believe that you can stand on your own two feet.

You just don't believe in yourself anymore, so you doubt every move you take. Actually, you stop making any moves at all because you are waiting for other people to tell you what to do. You're afraid you'll make a mistake.

Having the power to make your own decision and having your life back for you to decide can be very scary.

The fear of failure and feelings of incompetence consumes us and we are unable to make any decision without going into a complete panic attack.

I remember vividly how I was very critical and doubtful of my own abilities. I felt so much pressure to hold it all together and do well for me and my daughter. I also felt like I was crumbling, negative thoughts clouded my mind: "I am inferior, I am not capable, and who is going to hire me? I am not smart enough to go back to school"

I was very anxious and nervous of falling flat on my face, of proving him right that I couldn't make it on my own, that was useless. That's when I decided that I needed to talk to somebody about what happened. I needed to understand and get these words out of my head. I needed to talk.

After meditating a lot and talking about this with my family and a therapist, I earned a little bit of understanding and confidence in myself. Enough to make me want to get up and start fighting for my life.

While talking about what I went through with the domestic violence and emotional abuse, I started to realize something about my past that became a crucial starting point in my recovery.

I realized that before I was in such a chaotic relationship, I was happy. I was successful; I had a great career, great friends, and a great social life. People wanted my advice, my knowledge, and my friendship. I was standing on my own two feet before I met him, and best of all, I was happy back then, before him.

How can I go back to the old me that I missed so much? How can I go back to feeling fulfilled and like my old self again?

The answer came to me as fast as I could think it, all I had to do was go back to what made me happy: my hobbies, my passions, doing the things that made me feel fulfilled.

It was not going to be easy though, being oppressed and be littered for so long had erased my own sense of self. I had forgotten what do I like? What are my passions? What makes me happy?

I had been unhappy and forgotten for so long that I was lost in my own world. However, I had a slither of hope that I was going to find them again.

That little bit of hope that I was able to pull from deep within me, was the spark that ignited my own pursuit of happiness. I was going to get back to that happy place, and I was going to fight to stay there.

Positive Thoughts

I started to repeat positive thoughts and affirmations about myself. When things got tough, I would replace negative thoughts like "this is too hard", to "this is a challenge, I can do this".

I began to actually feel an appreciation for my strength. I was proud that I was out there making it and killing it! I got a great job, graduated from college. I bought a car, had a nice condo. Life was looking good so far!

Belief is the enemy of the doubt. Learn to think positively and believe in your ability to be successful. Remember you will succeed if you think you will and you will fail if you think that too. Your thoughts are self-fulfilling prophecies so you really have to try to reverse negative thoughts.

That is what an abusive relationship will do to you. It will make you doubt anything you think and any decision you make. Take the power back by allowing yourself to go ahead and make a mistake if you have to. Life is about learning and growing, falling down and getting back up. You have to keep moving forward.

How to Overcome Self-Doubt

1. **Stop Negativity on its tracks**
   Don't let your thoughts get out of control, stop them at their tracks. Talk to yourself, "you're not going to sabotage yourself!" Stop the thought pattern and it won't take over.

2. **Talk**
   Refer to your support system to just talk it out. Sometimes expressing our thoughts out loud to someone we trust can put things back into perspective. If that person is supportive of you and your efforts, you can gain valuable insight that will propel you forward into your goals.

3. **Stop Comparing**
   Never compare yourself to others, you never know what they had to go through to get where they are. Their lives are not your life. Only compare yourself to yourself, your life and struggles, your successes and failures. Compare your life before with your life now.

4. **Setbacks are temporary**
   If you have a failure it can quickly send you back to doubting every decision you make. Just think that it is normal to fail from time to time. See it as an opportunity to learn, and get back up. It's easy to use this setback as an excuse to not take

action. Learn from your mistakes and keep on moving forward.

5. **Celebrate any small success**
   No matter how big or small, a win is a win. Celebrate all your milestones and treat yourself. Finally got that job you wanted? Buy your favorite meal from that restaurant you like. Celebrating all your victories will keep you motivated, and will give you the strength to fight that self-doubt and move forward towards achieving your goals.

6. **Avoid negative people**
   If there somebody in your new life that is discouraging and negative, especially when it comes to you, get rid of them. Yes, even family. Always be in the company of those people whose thoughts and attitudes toward life, in general, are positive.

> *"Our doubts are traitors, and make us lose the good we oft might win, by fearing to attempt."*
> **William Shakespeare**

Chapter 10.
Never stop doing this

Leaving an abusive relationship can leave you really wiped out. You are emotionally drained; it's hard to think clearly when you have so much to do. It's hard to just stop and come out with a plan, but the truth is, without a plan you are not going to get anywhere far, or anywhere worth going.

It's time to keep working on yourself to become a better version of you. Enhance our strengths, and improve our weaknesses. It's time to break bad habits and become selfish with our time and our efforts. This is the time to rebuild, and you need every bit of energy you can find in yourself.

I have compiled my best tips on how you can improve yourself every day. Some of these can be implemented right away, some make take some planning. They are all worth trying, and if you are afraid to step out of your comfort zone, that's because it's a shot worth taking.

Here are the tips:

   1. **Read books**

As I became passionate about self-improvement, I began to read books by those famous gurus and gained so much valuable insight. Every time I read a page that spoke to me, I felt such a relief that I wasn't alone in my pain. That it was ok to feel bad sometimes and have bad days. It's getting up and trying your best that counts.

Visit your local library and pick up some books to read, check out the Self-Help section or Psychology.

2. Get Creative

Doing something that makes you happy, and let you be creative and have fun, can make wonders for your self-steam and lower your stress.

It's never too late to pick up an Easel, or if you fancy woodworking, knitting, jewelry making. There are so many things you can do, even if small, that can bring joy into your life.

All you have to do is ask yourself, what do you enjoy doing? Even if it's just sitting watching a movie or documentary, do it every day even if for a few minutes.

3. Take a class

Check your local college or online school and register for a course. Maybe a cooking class, writing or special topics like history or music, can really bring back some happiness into your life.

Plus, you will have the chance to meet new people, some will share your same interests and will give you an opportunity to clear your mind and feel relaxed.

4. Create an exercise routine

Even if it's just a brisk walk after dinner or a stroll through the park twice a week, make it a point to get out there and move your body!

Not only will it help you to get in better physical shape, but it will also lower your stress, and help you clear your mind. If you're also dealing with anger issues or outbreaks, running or playing sports can help alleviate those angry feelings.

5. Create Lists

If you have your goal in front of you, with the steps necessary to achieve it, there is a better chance that you will complete and succeed, than if you just leave it to your brain to remember.

Creating lists can help you be more productive, as you can go through your list the moment you feel lost and don't know what to do next.

6. Quit a Bad habit

If you've been meaning to quit smoking, lose weight, oversleeping, or any other bad habit, this is the time to quit.

Talk to your doctor to make sure you are doing it correctly, and don't forget to celebrate your victory once you get rid of it.

7. Toxic people? Get rid of them

Everyone has that person or persons that are considered toxic. Those that do nothing but judge you and bring you down; it's time to get rid of them.

8. Start a Journal

Be honest and write from the heart. As you write and you read it back, you will gain valuable insight about your feelings, and you will be able to deal with issues more openly.

9. Check in with Yourself

It's easy to get into the hamster wheel of life and just go go go all the time. Taking the time to step back and look at your life, can help you understand what's going right, and what needs adjusting.

Ask yourself, Am I ok? Am I happy? Am I moving forward towards my goals? What do I need to change?

Write in your journal these questions and the answers, and you can find out where you need to work on.

10. Check in with the World

Put your phone away, go outside and sit in nature. Even if it's just a patch of grass, just close your eyes and enjoy the sun on your skin, the wind brushing against your hair, enjoy the smell of the earth. Check in with nature as often as you can, and give your mood a lift.

"If you always do what you've always done, you'll always be where you've always been." —*T.D. Jakes*

"Beginning today, set an intention and a relentless focus on living your life as the greatest person you can be, in all situations." —*Brendon Burchard*

"The dreaming has to be backed up by the doing." —*Carrie Wilkerson*

Chapter 11.
Retrain your brain

Something that I found really helpful, was teaching myself to stop thinking negatively, and instead, concentrate on what good and positive things were going on in my life. This way I was slowly retraining my brain to give me the boost I needed to keep moving forward and reaching my goals.

This was not an overnight process; I did experience some setbacks. Settling back into the negative ways that you probably have been used to for so long can be a hard habit to break. But it's very important that you become your best advocate, and allow your self-esteem to improve. You can only do that if you stop the negative thoughts.

That night when I decided to leave, I went back to bed but I couldn't sleep. My mind was racing and I was so anxious. I was going to get my life back and I was prepared to do whatever it took. I was getting out for good this time. I was about to take control of my life and this time, nobody is going to stop me or derail me.

I cut all contact, I got a restraining order and I made sure he knew I was serious about staying away. My life meant so much more to me now that I was going to be a mother. You have to take your life seriously in order for anyone to take you seriously as well.

Emotionally I was a complete wreck. I was basically terrified of the unknown. I was a complete mess of emotions.

I felt so worried, what was I going to do? I have to find a place to live, build a nursery. I have to increase my work hours, get my finances in order. I have no furniture, I have to get a new car because the one I have is too small for the baby.

I felt so overwhelmed because I had so much to do. But you know what? It felt so good to have my own plans again, I even caught myself smiling. Suddenly, I felt extremely hopeful and excited.

How to Retrain Your Brain

1. **Be mindful of your thoughts**.
   Are negative thoughts invading your mind sabotaging your progress? Whenever you start to feel negative and feel that heavy weight in your chest, be aware of your own thoughts, and realize that you have to start to think better of yourself.

2. **Use an App**
   Yep! There's an app for that. In this digital age, there is an app that will pop up and fill you up with positive vibes throughout the day. Head over to your app store, both iPhone and Android has extensive selections of affirmations apps, pick a few and try them out until you find the one that works for you.

3. **Turn a negative into a positive**
   Instead of saying "I can't lose weight, its helpless", say "I love my body, I am beautiful, and I will continue to

try my best to look my best." Stop getting in your own way, nobody is perfect, you try and try again until you make it.

4. **Meditation**
Find a quiet place to sit or lay down, start taking deep breaths and concentrating on your breathing. Concentrating on your body relaxing muscle by muscle. Imagine a ray of light coming through your breathing and illuminating your body from the inside out. Feel the calmness of the moment, feel the pressure just coming off you. It will take practice but once you get it, you'll have a clear mind.

5. **Focus on happiness**
Does finishing that crossword puzzle makes you happy? How about a little retail therapy? Volunteering or doing crafts? By focusing on what gives you joy; you will transform your sadness into happiness. Sometimes just enjoying something simple like a cup of coffee at your favorite place, can make all the difference. Write in your journal a list of these things, and try to do at least two each day.

6. **Keep on Moving**
It's no secret that physical exercise is great for the body and mind. So why not start? There is so much benefit that you can gain and your body will thank you. A simple brisk walk for 30 minutes after dinner can help you relax, lose weight, enjoy the world around

you, and just take your mind away from the everyday stresses. Bring the kids into it for an afternoon of exploration around your neighborhood.

Start to make plans again. Dig in your heart for your happiness, for your passion. Whatever your dreams might be, you can achieve anything if you make it a goal.

Lean on your strength, on the faith in yourself and embrace your fears. There is nothing better than making your own way, you can do it!

Affirmations are a really great way to retrain your brain to love yourself again. Embrace change and your new future, you deserve the best!

Affirmations to help you stay strong and embrace change.

1. I possess what I need to get through this.
   Feeling sorry for yourself and calling yourself a victim will only make you even more doubtful of your own abilities. Focus on what have: your courage, your willpower, and your worth.

2. Time heals all wounds
   What today seems like a mountain of pain and suffering is crushing on top of you; just know that in time, it will all pass. You will start to feel like yourself again; you just need to let time do its thing.

3. I am in control of my life, reactions, and feelings.
   How you react to what happens around you is your choice, you have to stop putting blame on others. Those who hurt you want you to react negatively, surprise them by creating positive changes in your life.

4. I must take care of myself first
   Helping others is a great way to feel good about yourself, but it won't help you if you are suffering as a consequence. Make sure you are in a good place in your life, before you help anyone do the same.

5. It's Okay if I fail, I can start again
   It's so easy to give up when there is an obstacle or failure. That's why many abused people go back to a dangerous situation. Success never comes easy, never be afraid to start again and again as many times as you need to until you succeed. You owe it to yourself.

6. I am ready for a change. I accept and love myself exactly as I am.
   There is only one of you; therefore you're perfect for you.

7. I trust myself, I create my own destiny.
   Your future looks great, keep working at it!

8. I face this challenge with strength and know that I will get through this.

You are stronger than you think, you will succeed.

9. I am stronger, wiser and more confident with each new day.

10. I now begin a project that will change my life forever – I am unstoppable!

About The Author

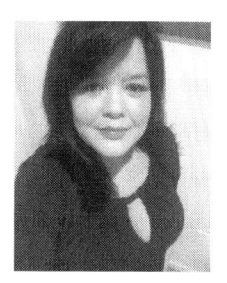

Gigi Rosa is a writer out of South Florida. She specializes in self-help and dating topics. As a survivor of domestic violence, her mission is to educate other women so they don't find themselves in another abusive relationship.

When she is not writing, educating or inspiring other women to succeed and live the life of their dreams, you can find her creating a recipe in the kitchen, or playing with her two kids.

Learn more about Gigi at http://www.safewhatnow.com/gigi_rosa/

One Last Thing...

If you enjoyed this book or found it useful, I'd be very grateful if you'd post a short review on Amazon. Your support really does make a difference and I read all the reviews personally, so I can get your feedback and make this book even better.

Thanks again for your support!

Printed in Great Britain
by Amazon